The Science is Settled!

Vaccines are safe.

The "Gold Standard" Randomized Double-Blind Placebo Controlled Unconflicted Research

Holly Garrison

ISBN-13:
978-1548595142

ISBN-10:
1548595144

DEDICATION

This book is dedicated to my children, Alex, Seth, Lance, and Layla. You have educated me more than any of my formal schooling. I love you more than you can imagine! You have filled my life with love and laughter, each equally important.

Mom

Introduction

My intention for writing this book is to start a conversation. It should not be mistaken for medical advice.

The topic of vaccine safety is hotly debated daily in professional settings as well as social media. We all hear the mainstream media's cry, "Vaccines are safe, vaccines are effective!" We hear this echoed throughout doctor's offices. We have heated debates in our various social media groups. The mantra, "The science is settled!" has been used on a variety of topics from DNA to climate change. But is it? Is science ever settled?

I became a mother in 2003 and began researching vaccinations, only after my twin sons were well into their first year of life. I did what most of us do. I listened diligently to my doctors through every test, induction, intervention, treatment, management, supplementation, and surgery. They were on schedule with their vaccinations and were participants in a study for a version of the flu mist vaccine. Some things went against my motherly instincts and I began to question every decision we had made. I began researching everything I could find on vaccines. Fast forward to today, my twins are almost 14, and I am now a mother to four beautiful and unique children.

I am also a chiropractor and practice near my hometown in West Virginia. Many patients ask my opinion about vaccinations. I have to tell them that professionally it is out of my scope of practice, therefore I cannot give them medical advice on this topic. However, I can direct them to resources and advise them to do their own research.

As a mom, I understand that not everyone is going to sit through 40 plus hours of documentaries on any topic. Most people don't have time to critically look at the information that is available, break down the study, and look up the authors' affiliations or conflicts. So, I decided to compile a list of the credible studies that passed muster when it came to following clinical trial research protocols. This included studies that had followed the "gold standard" of using a study design known as randomized double-blind placebo controlled, or RDBPC. To be included in this book, a study had to actually use a true placebo. A placebo is by definition: an inert, harmless, pill, medicine, or procedure that has no therapeutic effect. Secondly, a study also had to pass the sniff test and follow proper data analysis and stick to their original study design. A third criterion I used eliminated studies that had obvious conflicts of interest or affiliations of the lead scientists. In other words, these studies had to live up to the standards that are applied to every other industry for following proper research criteria, i.e. proper science. I also included the safety studies that were done on the number of vaccines children are required to have according to the CDC's recommended schedule or for school entrance.

The following pages are a summary of the studies that followed this criteria, can actually be called “science”, and therefore offer proof of the safety of vaccines and the way they are being implemented today.

The Science is Settled!

Intentionally Blank

Intentionally Blank

Intentionally Blank

Wait, wait, wait! By now you may have realized that most of this book is blank.

You may be thinking that you were duped. In honesty, by the industries own admission, almost no safety studies for vaccines use a true placebo. There are no studies on the safety of the recommended schedules. There are questions of fraud and malfeasance on every level.

It is my wish that you use this book to continue your own research into vaccine safety. Feel free to use these blank pages to take notes on your journey. It is also my wish that every parent be afforded the right to make choices for their own families, based on health history, personal beliefs, or religious faith. I initially did not list references as it would be nearly impossible to list all of the studies that I have read and evaluated over the years. However, my persistent brother-in-law, whom I solicited to be my first draft editor, suggested that the controversial and serious nature of this topic warranted some discussion and references. I hope, to his approval, that I have covered the topic succinctly enough to show that the science surrounding vaccine safety is most assuredly not settled. I welcome conversation and criticism. I would love to be proven inaccurate and be presented with a study on vaccine safety that does, in fact, fit the RDBPC model.

Please flip to page 121

The Science is Settled!

Intentionally Blank

Intentionally Blank

Intentionally Blank

Intentionally Blank

Intentionally Blank

Intentionally Blank

Intentionally Blank

Intentionally Blank

Intentionally Blank

Intentionally Blank

Intentionally Blank

Intentionally Blank

Intentionally Blank

Intentionally Blank

Intentionally Blank

Intentionally Blank

Intentionally Blank

Intentionally Blank

Intentionally Blank

Intentionally Blank

Intentionally Blank

Intentionally Blank

Intentionally Blank

Intentionally Blank

Intentionally Blank

Intentionally Blank

Intentionally Blank

Intentionally Blank

Intentionally Blank

Intentionally Blank

Intentionally Blank

Intentionally Blank

Intentionally Blank

Intentionally Blank

Intentionally Blank

Intentionally Blank

Intentionally Blank

Intentionally Blank

Intentionally Blank

Intentionally Blank

Intentionally Blank

Intentionally Blank

Intentionally Blank

Intentionally Blank

Intentionally Blank

Intentionally Blank

Intentionally Blank

Intentionally Blank

Intentionally Blank

Intentionally Blank

Intentionally Blank

Intentionally Blank

Intentionally Blank

Intentionally Blank

Intentionally Blank

Intentionally Blank

Intentionally Blank

Intentionally Blank

Intentionally Blank

Intentionally Blank

Intentionally Blank

Intentionally Blank

Intentionally Blank

Intentionally Blank

Intentionally Blank

Intentionally Blank

Intentionally Blank

Intentionally Blank

Intentionally Blank

Intentionally Blank

Intentionally Blank

Intentionally Blank

Intentionally Blank

Intentionally Blank

Intentionally Blank

Intentionally Blank

Intentionally Blank

Intentionally Blank

Intentionally Blank

Intentionally Blank

Intentionally Blank

Intentionally Blank

Intentionally Blank

Intentionally Blank

Intentionally Blank

Intentionally Blank

Intentionally Blank

Intentionally Blank

Intentionally Blank

Intentionally Blank

Intentionally Blank

Intentionally Blank

Intentionally Blank

Intentionally Blank

Intentionally Blank

Intentionally Blank

Intentionally Blank

Intentionally Blank

Intentionally Blank

Intentionally Blank

Intentionally Blank

Intentionally Blank

Intentionally Blank

Intentionally Blank

Intentionally Blank

Intentionally Blank

Intentionally Blank

Intentionally Blank

Intentionally Blank

A note from the author

I recognize that a portion of readers are typical American parents that are overwhelmed by the contradictory information that we hear daily. They may not take it upon themselves to look at any references listed at the back of this book or any other resource. Of the ones that do, how many will be able to decipher the medical jargon? Therefore, I find it relevant to discuss the references I included in this text as a way to show just how convoluted and unsettled the science really is. Again, this is not to be taken as medical advice. This book is not intended to be used as a substitute for self-education. It is merely an avenue to continue the debate, and give a voice to those who have not been heard.

I come from a region known as Appalachia, or more specifically, West Virginia, where many are undereducated, compared to the national average, according to the Appalachian Regional Commission. (24) Note I say "undereducated", not uneducated.

It is important to mention Mississippi here as well. According to the U.S. education department, Mississippi's post secondary education and graduation rates are lower than the national average. (20)

Why do I bring up West Virginia and Mississippi exclusively? West Virginia and Mississippi have some of the highest vaccine rates in the nation according to the CDC. (25) Unfortunately, both states also have some of the highest infant mortality rates. (19) I am not claiming causation. I am just noting some facts and praying that the policy makers and professionals will take it upon themselves to solve this problem. It should not be safer to have a baby in Cuba or South Korea than it is in West Virginia. It should not be safer to have a baby in Bahrain than in Mississippi. *Something is rotten in the state of Denmark* but it is safer to have a baby there. (16) (7)

I also want to shine a light on the fact that the only two states that have never had religious or philosophical vaccine exemptions are also the states with the lowest number of citizens with college degrees. Many of the people from these regions that do gain a college education tend to leave and find employment and better opportunities for themselves and their families. (14) I will leave it to the reader to draw a conclusion about a connection between under-education, poverty, and rights violations.

Some of the families that are looking for answers and asking for reform in vaccine policy from my region lack: a higher education, the training necessary to read and understand research, the confidence to stand up for their rights, and the ability to make an informed decision. This same lack comes into play in the voting booth. If we don't understand the issues or even know what rights are guaranteed to us in the United States Constitution and our state constitutions, how can we make an informed decision? When electing public officials, how are we to differentiate, those that would be responsible for standing up for the rights of their citizens? How are we to hold them accountable when they fail. Especially, if we don't even notice…

Many of the people I have joined forces with are in fact amongst the most highly educated professionals in the state. We have among the freedom fighters in West Virginia; medical doctors, pharmacists, chiropractors, lawyers, naturopaths, midwives, researchers, public officials, and parents from every walk of life. Many of us have nothing in common, and had never met, until we or someone we loved experienced a health crisis. Some of us have never experienced this personally but understand that giving up any personal right for the greater good, is a slippery slope. Some of us have no "skin in the game" (so to speak), but got involved out of a sense of duty. A sense that as an educated individual it is our responsibility to stay in West Virginia and fight for the rights of everyone living within her geographically isolated borders. Many of these warriors have literally put their livelihoods on the line, in order to stand up for the rest of us.

Discussion

Placebo

This book was originally designed to be completely blank, but given the serious nature of the topic I have been asked to include a few references. First I would point out that the vaccine industry freely admits that they do not use true, inert placebos. An article published by the World Health Organization, WHO, discusses the rationale behind why they do not use true placebos in vaccine trials. (11) In short, the claim is, that having a true control or using a real placebo is unethical because it would withhold potentially life-saving interventions from one group of participants. However, they not only use prior versions of vaccines that were previously "approved by the FDA as safe" and completely different vaccines as placebos, they also use shots of an aluminum adjuvant as a placebo. (10) I am not sure how giving a shot of aluminum or a placebo that contains polysobate 80, yeast, and other potentially reactive components of a vaccine is considered a life-saving intervention. Yet that is exactly what they did in the Gardasil (HPV or Human Papillomavirus) trials. (31)

An article in *The Lancet*, discusses the availability of true placebos to independent researchers, stating, "Independent researchers might end up compromising—or even abandoning—their research design because of the unwillingness of some pharmaceutical companies to deliver placebo drugs or devices. We believe that this could be a major way for the pharmaceutical industry to control scientific information about their drugs." (4)

So we see that the vaccine industrial complex not only decides that it doesn't have to follow true clinical trial protocol, citing ethics, but can also throw those same ethics out the window, whenever the manufacturer decides to. Consequently, if the ethical argument of not using a placebo can be thrown out and safety data is still accepted and validated then the excuse used by the WHO, is just that, an excuse.

The WHO article on placebo use says, "However, there are several examples demonstrating that a vaccine that is effective in one population is not always equally effective in others. The vaccine may have been developed for strains of viruses/ bacteria different from those that exist in the target population in the LMIC (low middle income countries) (e.g. conjugate pneumococcal vaccines). There may also be genetic, epidemiological, demographic or environmental differences affecting the target population that modify the efficacy of the vaccine (e.g. rotavirus vaccines)." (10)

Yet, the CDC and DHHR insist on mandating these vaccines and recommending these vaccines to everyone regardless of nationality, race, "demographics", family medical history, and a host of other individual, relative data that could help doctors identify a person's risk of developing a severe reaction.

Another good resource is the actual package insert from the manufacturer of each vaccine. An eye opening amount of information can be found there. For example this is a quote from a package insert for a leading vaccine, "Because clinical trials are conducted under widely varying conditions, adverse event rates observed in the clinical trials of a vaccine cannot be directly compared with rates in the clinical trials of another vaccine, and may not reflect the rates observed in practice." (17) This vaccine trial was conducted using statistics from a former version of a similar vaccine, not a true, inert placebo. So when they say safe, what they mean is "safe, compared to another vaccine" or "safe, compared to a toxic adjuvant injection."

I think I am secure in stating that most of the studies on vaccine safety do not follow RBDPC protocols. Most studies do not use true, inert, placebos. Therefore how can we say that the science is settled? How can we say that vaccines are safe, in a declarative sentence without qualifiers? The definition of safe is: not exposed to danger or risk. When the safety data shows many reactions, including death, we are in fact being exposed to risk. Therefore, it would be accurate to say, " this vaccine is as safe as other vaccines." But to make blanket statements about safety is flawed. Based on the current evidence, all vaccines are not safe for everyone.

Herd Immunity

"Well what about the greater good?" you ask. I will direct you to a good article on the topic by Dr, Russell Blaylock, *The Deadly Impossibility of Herd Immunity Through Vaccination.* (3)

It is significant that 57 other states in the US have exemption laws and there are no epidemics breaking out, as a result, despite the media magnifying small outbreaks. Let's take the case of measles in Minnesota. According to news outlets, several online publications (and my own hometown newspaper) "75 cases were reported in a state with a population of 5.5 million people." That is less than one percent and there were no deaths (as of this writing) associated with these cases. (18)

Just to briefly address this, let me explain that the Samli community in Minnesota was seeing a higher percentage of autism rates and therefore started skipping the MMR (measles, mumps, and rubella) shot. (27) Refer back to the WHO paper that discussed why all vaccines may not be as effective for different populations. I would extrapolate that they also may not be as safe for all demographics, races, or people of various origins.

Another article of note is a study by Jason M. Warfel, et al., discussing the growing number of whooping cough (pertussis) cases despite high vaccination rates. (31) The study stated that vaccinated individuals could still contract, carry, and spread pertussis, even if they were asymptomatic. So claiming that "mandatory vaccine laws are made to protect public health and stop the spread of communicable disease" isn't always the end result. To put this in layman's terms, we have created a population of "pertussis Marys" (look up typhoid Marys if this is lost on you). I will not go into the concept of "shedding" but essentially live viruses in vaccines can be "shed" or transmitted to others for a certain period of time following vaccinations. (2)

I will also say that in a perfect world all vaccines would be attenuated (weakened) or killed to the point of not causing disease or "shedding". Are vaccine manufactures not subjected to human error? Is it possible that "bad batches" can happen? Has it happened? This is a topic for another book as well. I will say the words, "Tennessee, bad batches, and dead babies." and leave this topic like a mystery for you to solve on your own.

Combination Shots

Another important point about pertussis is that we no longer are offered individual vaccinations for pertussis. The current vaccines have five different viruses or virus components in it including; diphtheria, tetanus, pertussis (whooping cough), hepatitis B, and poliomyelitis. This is important because the multivalent (containing more than one virus or virus component) vaccines have a more controversial history in the safety department. In a study done in 1986 by Javier Sedarait, they gave mice an injection of vaccine A and they were fine. (15) Then they gave mice a shot of vaccine B and they were fine. Then they gave the mice a shot of vaccine A and B in the same injection and many of the mice died. There is a lot of complicated mumbo jumbo about how the viruses used did some kind of scary dance and recombined to form a more invasive virus that penetrated the brain and spinal cord of the dead mice. They used the term "neuroinvasive".

However, I should note that later in 1988, shortly after the laws changed to give vaccine manufacturers complete immunity from liability, these same authors took it upon themselves to redo the study, with the following findings: "It was found that, although neuroinvasive recombinant viruses could be detected in the spinal cords of the infected animals, most of the viruses (both recombinants and no recombinants) isolated from all tissues tested were nonneuroinvasive (i.e., no mice died as a result of footpad infection with high doses of such plaque-purified isolates). As a result of these findings, we propose that the virulence of the virus mixture is a consequence of the complementation as well as the generation and selection of neuroinvasive recombinants in spinal cords of these mice." (26)

Again, this is an example of a lot of mumbo jumbo saying, what, exactly? You would almost have to have a Ph.D. in biology or some other such field to even interpret what they heck they are saying. So, in this case, the science wasn't settled. I was only made aware of these studies when I attended an IPAK (The Institute for Pure and Applied Knowledge is a not-for-profit organization) conference in Pittsburg, Pennsylvania, earlier this year. I heard one of the speakers bring up one of these studies and I was flabbergasted that this information has been around since I was a little girl.

To clarify this a little more gently, A is fine, B is fine, A+B equals death (maybe, but we don't know why). They first thought it was the components of two nonneuroinvasive viruses that formed a recombinant virus which was neuroinvasive. To explain it is necessary to define the word recombinant.

A recombinant virus is a virus produced by recombining pieces of DNA using recombinant DNA technology. This may be used to produce viral vaccines or gene therapy vectors. It is also used to refer to naturally occurring recombination between virus genomes in a cell infected by more than one virus strain.(23) In other words, viruses have the ability to get into a cell and recombine into a totally new virus, which could be more virulent than the original components. In the first study, it was determined that this new recombined virus was the cause of death of these mice.

In the second study they declare that, while they did find these recombined neuroinvasive viruses, they couldn't possibly be what killed the mice. However, the authors failed to determine, disclose, or answer, "What did kill the mice, then?"

So let's do the math again. A is fine, B is fine, C is safe compared to A, D is only slightly worse than B (but not statistically significant when we skew the data to exclude the numbers we didn't like). So now the math is A+B+C+D= what? There are no studies on the multivalent vaccinations that constitute most of what is on the market today. There are no studies on giving a child multiple shots, each containing multivalent vaccines, on one day. Again I will be happy if someone can correct the previous two statements.

But let's just sweep it under the rug, that we have known for the better part of 30 years, that multivalent vaccines present more of a risk and keep moving forward making more and more vaccines with more and more viruses in them.

There are now pentivalent (that's five viruses as mentioned above) and hexavalent (that's six) and many, many more X-valent vaccines on the market and "in the pipeline" as I am told by several experts I have heard speak at conferences I attended. You can search for yourself on the World Health Organization's website. (33)

MMR, Autism, and CDC Fraud

Lastly and most notoriously, in the multivalent vaccine drama, is the MMR. This came under fire in 1998 when Dr. Andrew Wakefield et al. published a paper in a British medical journal called *The Lancet*, raising a concern about the MMR vaccine and linking it to gastrointestinal issues. While it is known that gastrointestinal issues are often a co-morbidity with autism, Dr. Wakefield and his co-authors did not say that the MMR caused autism. I have cited *The Lancet* many times throughout this section since *The Lancet* article triggered the beginning of the attempted ruination of Dr. Wakefield. He has been the subject of and poster child for the powers that be to "debunk" a link between MMR and autism. This topic is worthy of many books and investigation on its own. To be succinct, Dr. Wakefield was "debunked" and then his "debunking" was "debunked". In essence there is a lot of BUNK involved in vaccine research, in speaking out about vaccines, or even asking questions. (6) Dr. Wakefield may or may not have had conflicts of interest. Dr. Wakefield did or did not follow protocol when he collected samples from children's colons and found measles virus growing there. Even if Dr. Wakefield had conflicts and didn't follow proper protocol (by doing colonoscopies on children with autism which wasn't considered medically necessary at the time). No one disputed that he found measles growing in these children's guts.

The over turning of the Wakefield case is another good example of "settled science" not being entirely settled. This is especially important considering the MMR is also the subject of the 2004 study that is quoted time and time again as proof that the MMR doesn't cause autism. (8)

This study has now surpassed the Wakefield study in notoriety, because it has come under fire after a whistleblower at the CDC was involuntarily "outed" and advised to file for whistleblower status for self-protection. If you look at the authors of this study you will see W Thompson listed. A further search of "William Thompson CDC whistle blower" produces multiple sources showing that evidence of outright fraud on the part of the CDC has been given to congress. To date, we wait with baited breath for Thompson's subpoena to testify before congress. (9) There are also articles dismissing William Thompson's evidence and the man that brought forth the information, Dr. Brian Hooker. Accusations that there was no evidence of fraud and subsequently the MMR study should be considered valid, overlook a few important facts. Either the researchers were instructed to falsify data and destroy evidence which completely invalidates this study; or one of the lead researchers that was responsible for data analysis, is a total crack pot which again totally invalidates this study. Again "settled science?" I don't think this qualifies.

Two other players of significance in this investigation are the lead author of this study, Frank Destefano and the head of the CDC during this study and subsequent alleged fraud, Julie Gerberding.

First Frank Destefano is a renowned scientist and author employed at the CDC. He has been out spoken about the safety of thimerosal *(a mercury-based* preservative) in vaccines. (22) Even though the CDC and other studies suggest that thimerosal is safely eliminated from the body, "it was removed from most vaccines in 2001." (29) According to a study in 2005, there is evidence to suggest that the reason ethyl mercury in vaccines leaves the blood stream faster, is because it crossed the blood brain barrier and went into the brain tissue and other organs. The blood levels of ethyl mercury from thimerosal were not excreted from the body as the CDC website above still claims. This study suggests a much more serious need to study thimerosal and its effects on humans, which directly contradicts the "settled science" on thimerosal. (4)

Second, Julie Gerberding was the head of the CDC when Dr. Thompson allegedly contacted his superiors to notify them of the statistically significant data regarding MMR and autism. It is unclear if she knew about and ordered the fraud and cover up at the CDC. However, she no longer works for the CDC. Spoiler alert: she now has a six or seven figure salary working for BIG Pharma … Which Big Pharma company? You guessed it, the maker of one of the MMR vaccines, MERCK. (13) I don't know about you, but quite frankly, I smell a rat! (21)

In Closing

This book doesn't even scratch the surface on all the information on vaccines and safety issues. According to Tim Albury, author of *Reason if you will,*

"Settled Science" = Oxymoron (1)

A choice is really all most parents are seeking. If we had only been given a choice, we would have happily worked with our pediatrician and made the best decision for our families. Instead, we are called to action when our rights and the rights of those around us are being trampled on.

To quote Barbra Loe Fisher, co-author of *DPT: A Shot in the Dark*, and founder of the National Vaccine Information Center; "Where there is risk, there must be choice." (12)

Acknowledgements

I am now, quite willfully shirking all manner of decorum by placing this section at the end of the book. Otherwise, it would have given away the "gag" too soon. I would like to acknowledge the initial inspiration to write a book in this manner, Michael J. Knowles, author of *Reasons To Vote For Democrats: A Comprehensive Guide*. When you open this book, it too is blank, indicating that there is no reason to vote for democrats. I found this amusing and ingenious. That led me to other "gag" books authored by Rich Ferguson, which I studied as templates. However, in an effort to convey the seriousness of this topic I went rogue, and the results are the above creation.

I would also like to acknowledge the many people that inspired me to write this book:

I am awed at the tirelessness of Del Bigtree, Jimmy, and the entire Vaxxed team. Without the Vaxxed bus and the showing of Vaxxed here in WV, I would not have met so many amazing warriors that care, like me, about the fate of the children in our state.

Our team in West Virginia, without whom, I would not have found my voice; the members of West Virginians for Health Freedom. We are working day and night to increase vaccine risk awareness in our state. We have won and lost a battle or two, but have only just begun.

Many thanks to others that are involved with the vaccine risk awareness movement, safe vaccine movement, parental choice and health freedom movement. While there are too many to name these are just a few that I have met personally or have heard speak. Gratitude isn't an adequate word for many that have sacrificed careers and credibility to protect our children including: Robert Kennedy Jr., Dr. Sherri Tenpenny, Dr. Suzanne Humphries, Dr. Brian Hooker, Dr. Alvin Moss, and many other politicians, PhD's and medical doctors that have put their livelihoods and in some cases their vary lives on the line to expose the truth.

Matthew Loop, author of *Social Media Made Me Rich: Here's How it Can do the Same for You*, has inspired me as a colleague, a chiropractor, fellow alum, entrepreneur, author, guru, and an achiever beyond my comprehension. Thanks for fighting the good fight and all you do for our profession!

There were many teachers, mentors, and professors along the way that helped shape who I am today. Many of you pushed me outside of my comfort zone and helped me develop my ability to persevere.

My most humble appreciation to my family. Words fail to describe the support, guidance, and unconditional love they have given me. They inspire me daily to be my best self. Their support has allowed me to keep my feet on the ground and my head in the clouds. Eternal love!

Anyone that feels they have been left out of my acknowledgements, please consider yourself family…

With thanks to God and gratitude!

Holly

For more information about West Virginia's for Health Freedom and the progress we are making, please visit our website or find us on Facebook. https://www.facebook.com/groups/1059348450806623/

https://wvforhealthfreedom.com

The NVIC lists links to each states exemption laws, lists of the required vaccinations for school attendance, and updates on legislation. Please feel free to email me and I will send you an electronic version of the links and references in this text. www.nvic.org

If you would like to join me "down the rabbit hole," a good place to start is watching *Vaxxed*, or other documentaries including; *Vaccines Revealed*, *Trace Amounts, The Truth About Vaccines,* or *Direct Order.* Or just Google vaccine documentary and Netflix away.

References

1. Albury, Tim. "Settled Science" = Oxymoron." *"Settled Science" = Oxymoron*. N.p., 01 Jan. 1970. Web. 09 July 2017. http://www.reasonifyouwill.com/2014/03/settled-science-oxymoron.htm

2. Anderson, Evan J. "Rotavirus Vaccines: Viral Shedding and Risk of Transmission." The Lancet, Oct. 2008. Web. 09 July 2017. http://www.thelancet.com/journals/laninf/article/PIIS1473-3099(08)70231-7/fulltext.

3. Blaylock, Russell. "The Deadly Impossibility Of Herd Immunity Through Vaccination, by Dr. Russell Blaylock." *International Medical Council on Vaccination*. International Medical Council on Vaccination, 18 Feb. 2012. Web. 09 July 2017. http://www.vaccinationcouncil.org/2012/02/18/the-deadly-impossibility-of-herd-immunity-through-vaccination-by-dr-russell-blaylock/.

4. Burbacher, Thomas M., Danny D. Shen, Noelle Liberato, Kimberly S. Grant, Elsa Cernichiari, and Thomas Clarkson. "Comparison of Blood and Brain Mercury Levels in Infant Monkeys Exposed to Methyl mercury or Vaccines Containing Thimerosal." *Environmental Health Perspectives*. National Institute of Environmental Health Sciences, Aug. 2005. Web. 28 July 2017. https://www.ncbi.nlm.nih.gov/pmc/articles/PMC1280342/.

5. Christensen, Mikkel, and Filip K. Knop. "The Unobtainable Placebo: Control of Independent Clinical Research by Industry?" The Lancet, 7 Jan. 2002. Web. 09 July 2017. http://www.thelancet.com/journals/lancet/article/PIIS0140-6736(12)60024-5/fulltext?rss=yes

6. Crosby, Jake. "Lancet Keeps Wakefield Et Al. Retracted in Contempt of Court." *Autism Investigated*. N.p., 11 May 2014. Web. 09 July 2017. http://www.autisminvestigated.com/lancet-wakefield-retracted/

7. "COUNTRY COMPARISON: INFANT MORTALITY RATE." *Central Intelligence Agency*. Central Intelligence Agency, 2016. Web. 09 July 2017. https://www.cia.gov/library/publications/the-world-factbook/rankorder/2091rank.html,

8. DeStefano, F., T. K. Bhasin, W. W. Thompson, M. Yeargin-Allsopp, and C. Boyle. "Age at First Measles-mumps-rubella Vaccination in Children with Autism and School-matched Control Subjects: A Population-based Study in Metropolitan Atlanta." *Pediatrics.* U.S. National Library of Medicine, Feb. 2004. Web. 09 July 2017. https://www.ncbi.nlm.nih.gov/pubmed/14754936

9. Download The CDC Autism/MMR Files Released By Dr. William Thompson." *Vaxxed.* N.p., 26 Aug. 2016. Web. 09 July 2017. http://vaxxedthemovie.com/download-the-cdc-autism-mmr-files-released-by-dr-william-thompson

10. Exley, C. "Aluminium-based adjuvants should not be used as placebos in clinical trials." *Vaccine.* 2011;29:9289. Web. 09 July 2017. https://www.ncbi.nlm.nih.gov/pubmed/21871940.

11. "Expert Consultation on the Use of Placebos in Vaccine Trials." *WHO*. World Health Organization, 2013. Web. 09 July 2017. http://www.who.int/ethics/publications/9789241506250/en/

12. Fisher, Barbara Loe. "Your Health. Your Family. Your Choice." *National Vaccine Information Center (NVIC)*. N.p., 1982. Web. 09 July 2017. http://www.nvic.org/

13. "Former CDC Head Lands Vaccine Job at Merck." *Reuters*. Thomson Reuters, 21 Dec. 2009. Web. 09 July 2017. https://www.reuters.com/article/us-merck-gerberding-idUSTRE5BK2K520091221.

14. Jarvis, Jake. "Majority of WV Public College Grads Leave State for Work." *Charleston Gazette-Mail*. Staff Writer Charleston Gazette-Mail, 5 Nov. 2016. Web, 9 July 2017 http://www.wvgazettemail.com/news-education/20161105/majority-of-wv-public-college-grads-leave-state-for-work.

15. Javier RT, Sedarati F, Stevens JG. Two avirulent herpes simplex viruses generate lethal recombinants in vivo. *Science* 1986; 234: 746–748. Web 9 July 2017 https://www.ncbi.nlm.nih.gov/pubmed/3022376

16. Mabillard, Amanda. *Shakespeare Quick Quotes: Something is rotten in the state of Denmark. Shakespeare Online*. 20 Aug. 2010. Web. 9 July 2017 http://www.shakespeare-online.com//quickquotes/quickquotehamletdenmark.

17. "Manufacturer Package Insert." GlaxoSmithKline, 2016. Web. 09 July 2017 https://www.gsksource.com/pharma/content/dam/GlaxoSmithKline/US/en/Prescribing_Information/Pediarix/pdf/PEDIARIX.PDF

18. 2017, Michael Patrick Leahy 5 Jun. "Measles Outbreak Continues to Spread in Minnesota: 75 Cases Now Confirmed." *Breitbart*. N.p., 06 June 2017. Web. 09 July 2017. http://www.breitbart.com/big-government/2017/06/05/measles-outbreak-continues-to-spread-in-minnesota-75-cases-now-confirmed

19. National Center for Health Statistics. "Infant Mortality Rates by State." *Centers for Disease Control and Prevention*. Centers for Disease Control and Prevention, 04 Jan. 2017. Web. 09 July 2017. https://www.cdc.gov/nchs/pressroom/sosmap/infant_mortality_rates/infant_mortality.htm

20. "New State-by-State College Attainment Numbers Show Progress Toward 2020 Goal." Press Office, 12 July 2012. Web. 9 July 2017. https://www.ed.gov/news/press-releases/new-state-state-college-attainment-numbers-show-progress-toward-2020-goal

21. Online Dictionary and Translations. "*Online Dictionary and Translations*. N.p., n.d. Web. 09 July 2017. http://www.webster-dictionary.org

22. Price, Cristofer S., William W. Thompson, Barbara Goodson, Eric S. Weintraub, Lisa A. Croen, Virginia L. Hinrichsen, Michael Marcy, Anne Robertson, Eileen Eriksen, Edwin Lewis, Pilar Bernal, David Shay, Robert L. Davis, and Frank DeStefano. "Prenatal and Infant Exposure to Thimerosal From Vaccines and Immunoglobulins and Risk of Autism. "*Pediatrics*. American Academy of Pediatrics, 07 Sept. 2010. Web. 09 July 2017. http://pediatrics.aappublications.org/content/early/2010/09/13/peds.2010-0309

23. "Recombinant Virus." *Wikipedia*. Wikimedia Foundation, 10 Apr. 2017. Web. 09 July 2017. https://en.wikipedia.org/wiki/Recombinant_virus

24. Schwartz, Jeffrey H., Ed. D. "Development and Progress of the Appalachian Higher Education Network." *Executive Summary*. Appalachian Regional Commission, May 2004. Web. 09 July 2017. https://www.arc.gov/publications/DevelopmentandProgressoftheAHENetworkES.asp

25. Seither, Ranee, MPH, and Svetlana Masalovich, MS, et. al. "Vaccination Coverage Among Children in Kindergarten — United States, 2013–14 School Year." *Centers for Disease Control and Prevention*. Centers for Disease Control and Prevention, 17 Oct. 2014. Web. 09 July 2017. https://www.cdc.gov/mmwr/preview/mmwrhtml/mm6341a1.htm.

26. Sedarati, F., R. T. Javier, and J. G. Stevens. "Pathogenesis of a Lethal Mixed Infection in Mice with Two Nonneuroinvasive Herpes Simplex Virus Strains." *Journal of Virology*. U.S. National Library of Medicine, Aug. 1988. Web. 09 July 2017. https://www.ncbi.nlm.nih.gov/pubmed/2839719

27. Secretary, HHS Office of the, and Office For Civil Rights (OCR). "Summary of the HIPAA Privacy Rule." *HHS.gov*. US Department of Health and Human Services, 26 July 2013. Web. 09 July 2017. https://www.hhs.gov/hipaa/for-professionals/privacy/laws-regulations/index.html

28. "Study Finds High Rate of Autism among Minneapolis Somali Community." *Autism Speaks*. Federal Interagency Autism Coordinating, 24 July 2012. Web. 09 July 2017. https://www.autismspeaks.org/science/science-news/study-finds-high-rate-autism-among-minneapolis-somali-community.

29. "Vaccine Safety." *Centers for Disease Control and Prevention*. Centers for Disease Control and Prevention, 27 Oct. 2015. Web. 09 July 2017. https://www.cdc.gov/vaccinesafety/concerns/thimerosal/index.htm.

30. Vinton, Kate. "These 15 Billionaires Own America's News Media Companies." *Forbes*. Forbes Magazine, 02 June 2016. Web. 09 July 2017. https://www.forbes.com/sites/katevinton/2016/06/01/these-15-billionaires-own-americas-news-media-companies/#50c402a6660a

31. Warfel, Jason M., and Lindsey I. Zimmerman. "Jason M. Warfel." *Proceedings of the National Academy of Sciences*. National Acad Sciences, 22 Oct. 2013. Web. 09 July 2017. http://www.pnas.org/content/111/2/787.full

32. Winkel, Rich. "LACK OF DISCLOSURE OF "PLACEBO" INGREDIENTS IN CLINICAL TRIALS." *Thought Crime Radio*. N.p., 19 Aug. 2012. Web. 09 July 2017. http://thoughtcrimeradio.net/2012/08/lack-of-disclosure-of-placebo-ingredients-in-clinical-trials/

33. "WHO Vaccine Pipeline Tracker." *World Health Organization*. World Health Organization, June 2017. Web. 09 July 2017. http://www.who.int/immunization/research/vaccine_pipeline_tracker_spreadsheet/en/

For a digital copy of these references email me at

hollyg4vaxchoice@gmail.com

www.ingramcontent.com/pod-product-compliance
Lightning Source LLC
Chambersburg PA
CBHW031055180526
45163CB00002BA/851
9781548595142